Cut It Out!

Michael Kibler

DEDICATION

Dedicated to my love, Emily, who was there for me
every step of my journey.

CONTENTS

BACKGROUND

This is the story of my journey in which I found myself in the throes of an overwhelming addiction. My life was a wreck during high school. I was in special education for 4 years when I was younger due to severe ADHD, which set me back several years socially. Once my ADHD was under control, I was moved into a gifted program. Then, several years later, I skipped the eighth grade because I was too advanced for my current grade. Thus I entered high school at a severe social disadvantage. Even by the end of my senior year, I still struggled to be accepted by my peers. Kids can be very cruel to those that are different from them and I was no exception. I was a lost, confused, and enormously scared teenager that found myself among 2000 others who would not accept the person that I was. I was definitely not starting out on a good note.

And, on top of all that, I also had family problems. My father was a raging alcoholic who was tearing my family apart. He died of an overdose of alcohol and pain medications when I was very young. Even though my family life was stable by the time I entered high school, the ghosts of my past still continued to haunt me well into when I first tried what would become a terrible addiction

In my desperation to fit in at the time, and with the maturity brought about by puberty, I also yearned for a girlfriend. Finding a relationship drove me for most of my teenage years. I was obsessed with finding someone who would love me like I wanted to love them. Being that I was not that widely liked in school, I dated any girl who would take me. As a result, I was constantly in and out of abusive and unhealthy relationships which hindered my emotional and mental advancement. I was cheated on by my relationships on a regular basis and most of my girlfriends only kept me for up to a month. Not having any stability in my life translated into minimal stability for my emotional and mental states. This lack of concreteness in my life would end up hurting me in what was to be a very rough high school career.

Now I dated a girl when I was in high school who would cut herself. One day she told me that I should do it; that it "really helps" with life's problems. At this point in my life all I wanted was a lasting relationship, regardless of whether it was good for me or not; I wanted to please my partner so badly that I was willing to do quite nearly anything she told me to do. So I went into the bathroom with a knife and, by doing so, started my two year long addiction with cutting. Cutting soon began to run my entire life; the pain was electrifying, the highs were enthralling, and my addiction was ever-worsening. I couldn't go a single day without taking a razor blade to my wrist. My arm became a spider web of red scars. To see my blood running down my wrist brought about a sensation greater than any other I had ever felt. It wasn't that I was particularly depressed (though I did have the occasional bouts with depression); the simple fact of that matter was that it felt good to cut.

At first, I felt very guilty whenever I cut. I was ashamed of myself, which would make me cut even more. But eventually I got so wrapped up in my addiction that I didn't even care anymore. I distinctly remember several times I cut just for the sake of cutting. It was awful. I had an emotional attachment to the blade that surpassed everything else. My whole day revolved around when I could be alone with my razor. On school days I would ask to go to the restroom several times a day just to cut myself. I got to a point where I did not care about what people thought about my addiction; as long as I could cut, I was happy.

Yet I was not happy. While it is true that I was constantly medicating myself with the blade which gave others the impression that I was happy, I was, in no way, shape, or form, happy. I was slowly falling apart on the inside. I remember several times where I would have to slit my wrist just to keep from killing myself. I tremble to recall how close to the face of death I truly was on a regular basis. Deep down in the recesses of my subconscious, I knew that I was dying a miserable death. A death characterized by a tortuous addiction that lunged for my soul with every cut and scar I made. No person of this earth can really be happy when the source of the happiness is pain and suffering. It's just not in our design. We are made to be happy and rejoice in the company of others, not to isolate ourselves from everyone. And we are certainly not made to hurt ourselves. Not only does it go against our survival instincts, but it also goes against morality. This is why I felt so guilty when I first started cutting. However it is such a powerful addiction that from the moment I made my first cut, I was completely and utterly hooked on self harm.

As far as the actual cutting went, I was very "safe." I would always sterilize my blade before I cut, I never cut deep, and I always used my dominant hand to cut so I would have the most control I could. Needless to say, I did not have a death wish. I neither wanted, nor tried, to kill myself with cutting. Regardless, it was a vicious habit that had to end. All it took was one slip of my hand for the blade to hit an artery and I would have bled out in seconds, not to mention all the internal damage I was inflicting on myself.

I was hospitalized twice for various reasons including cutting. While the help they gave me was appreciated, it was not enough for me to stop. It wasn't until I made the commitment to myself to stop that I truly quit. And while the physical scars may be fading, I will always carry about the memories of a terrifyingly powerful addiction. There are still times in my life when I consider relapsing. But, with the tools and strategies I have outlined in this book, I am able to overcome the urges and live a better, healthier, and happier life. My hope is to impart the same tools and strategies to anyone struggling with any sort of self harm addiction.

WHAT IS SELF HARM AND WHY

Self harm, or self injury, is when a person deliberately inflicts pain or damage on themselves, often for therapeutic or cathartic purposes. Self harm is usual not done with the intent to kill one's self. It can be done in a variety of ways. The common ones are cutting, burning, biting, and scratching. No matter how it is done, self harm is a legitimate and very unhealthy addiction.

At first thought, for those fortunate ones who have not self harmed, this practice seems very counterintuitive. Why would you use pain to make yourself feel better? Why is something that hurts so addictive?

It all has to do with endorphins. In short, endorphins are a chemical produced by the body that cause feelings of pleasure and happiness. They are released during several different activities including sex, exercise, and, most importantly for the purposes of this book, pain. When an individual is in pain, endorphins are released to regulate that pain. And just as a person can get addicted to prescription pain killers, so too can a person get addicted to the body's natural pain killers, endorphins. So it is not the pain that people get hooked on, rather it is the body's natural defense against pain that gets them addicted.

There is another aspect of self harm that must be understood; control. An individual needs to be in complete control of their self harm in order to gain any relief from this vice. Whether it by razor blade or soldering iron, the person must be able to control and predict the exact moment of pain in order to feel any release from the pain. Humans, as a species, hate intermittent things, be it pain or sound or anything. If we can't predict it, we don't like it. That is why a person who cuts themselves five times a day often dreads going to the doctor's once a year to get a flu shot. That is also what separates self harm from masochism; masochists like the pain itself, but self harmers derive pleasure from the high that the pain causes the body to experience.

There is also a difference between self harming and other types of activities such as tattooing, piecing and religious fasting. These activities are not done for therapeutic purposes while self harm is done for that reason. Tattooing and piecing is, for the most part, strictly decorative or sentimental. Religious fasting is done for spiritual cleansing and is designed to be uncomfortable to the undertaker. Now there are those who argue that decorative self harm, or carving, is no different than tattooing and piercing. Rest assured that they are very different from each other. Tattooing and the likes are done for ornamental reasons, while self harm is done to hide from problems that an individual is facing. The only commonality between them is that they are destructive to the body, but for different reasons. And there are such things as excessive and even addictive tattooing and piercing. Any sort of addiction is a negative thing no matter how much of a positive thing the object of the addiction is. Too much of a good thing is still too much.

Just as I was not trying to commit suicide when I self harmed, most individuals who self harm do not do so to kill themselves. Usually it is the opposite; most people self harm to keep sane. It acts as a release to keep stress and angst from building up inside of them. However there are still dangers to any form of self harm no matter how safe the individual is. Infections, nerve damage, bleeding out, permanent scarring, and other damages can await those who practice self harm. There is also evidence that shows that there are a high percentage of people who self harmed within the percentage of people who have committed suicide. This means that those who self harm might be at a higher risk for attempting suicide. What the individual must realize is that there are healthier, safer, and more effective ways to deal with their problems than self harming. In effect, once the individual is done with the healing and learning processes, they will no longer have any reason to self harm.

In fact, most individuals only self harm severe enough to create a recognizable wound, however superficial it may be.

When I was cutting I would only cut deep enough to draw blood. As soon as I saw my own blood I would stop that particular cut. Let's call this the blood effect. Most self harmers hold true to the blood effect. Simply put, it is a self preservation method. When certain people see their own blood, their blood pressure drops and they become faint. I distinctly remember a time when I was having my blood drawn for testing and I glanced at my arm which they were taking the blood from and I literally blacked out for 30 seconds. This is called hemophobia. I believe we all have varying degrees of this fear of blood within ourselves to give us a healthy respect of injuries and to help us avoid injuring ourselves. I also believe this is what stops most individuals from self harming past a certain point. Remember that they are not trying to commit suicide; they are looking for relief. So it only makes sense that most individuals will stop a specific injury before that injury gets too severe.

Depression can have a lot to do with self harm. If an individual has more reasons to practice self harm, there is a greater chance that they will attempt it. That is why depression and self harm are usually so closely associated; depression, for the most part, enables the self harm and the self harm, in turn, reinforces the depression. It is a vicious cycle that must be broken in order to experience freedom and a happier life. Unfortunately, ridding the individual of the depression does not always guarantee that they quit self harming. I still experienced the urge to cut myself even when I had been clean for several months. It all depends on the individual as everyone is different. Finding out as much as possible about the individual can help to decode what drives them to self harm and how to get them to stop.

An individual can start self harming for a multitude of reasons. What started my first cutting episode was a combination of things. As I said earlier, my girlfriend at the time was encouraging me to try it. But it wasn't until I heard a song that glorified cutting and other self deprecating habits that I actually tried it. I was also under a lot of stress from school and my lack of a social life at the time which partially contributed towards my self harm battle. Usually there is more than one thing that triggers a person to start self harming. It doesn't have to be anything obvious to an observer. I know there were people a lot worse off than I was at the time, but it did not matter to me because I was looking inward and I did not care about the troubles of others. As far as I was concerned, I was the only one going through hard times. Those who self harm usually do not put things into proper perspective. As long as it is significant to them, then it is both real and important to the individual. Looking only inwardly for the most part is very unhealthy and will not accomplish much in the individual's life. The reason many self harmers do focus on inwardly on the negative is usually because they are trying to escape from the negatives by looking within. The actual problem is not in the negative aspects of the individual's life; it is how they view themselves and their environments. Teaching the individual how to look at the positive aspects of life can really make a difference on the path to healing.

In my experiences, there are two main triggers that work in conjunction with each other to start a person self harming; popular culture and relationships. Let's discuss popular culture first. For the most part, people today are surrounded by many bad examples, including that of self harming. The most common example is music. When I used to cut myself, I would normally listen to songs about cutting to enhance the experience. There are countless songs out there which present the idea, if not encourage, the notion of self harming. It is this kind of popular culture that embeds the idea of self harm in a person's mind. That is where relationships take over. If a given person is close to someone who does self harm, that person is more likely to try self harming and get addicted to it just through exposure. In short, popular culture plants the seed of self harm, and relationships can grow it.

Before I carried out an average episode, I would be extremely anxious and depressed. I craved the blade; I yearned for it. I would do nearly anything to be alone for long enough to carry out the deed. As soon as that blade went into my skin, all that anxiety and depression and bad thoughts would melt away into euphoria. I would feel like I was on the top of the world. Nothing could touch me; I was invincible. Any problem in my life became irrelevant. No matter what issues were invading my mind, I could escape from them. And if nothing was bothering me at the time, all the more better; it would boost my emotional status from normal to ecstatic. All I cared about was the sensation brought about by cutting. This high would last me for usually several hours unless I was having a particularly stressful day, in which case I would need to cut more often. I was medicating myself with pain; whenever I needed a pick-me-up, I'd go somewhere by myself and take another dose of pain. This describes most of my personal episodes. No doubt many out there feel the same way I did when they self harm. It is hard for those who have never self harmed to understand how it feels. But those who have know perfectly well what I'm talking about.

To give an idea of how many people really do engage in self harm, about 1% of the US population reported self harming. That might not seem like a lot, but it adds up to around 3 million people who reported engaging in self harm. That does not even cover all of those who hide their addiction, as most individuals do. So if you or someone you know self harms, know that you are not alone; there are millions out there with the same vice. Also know that help is available and things will always get better.

Some believe that self harm is just a phase or a temporary vice that will go away with time. This is a false belief. I know of people who have self harmed for upwards of 30 years and still engage in it. Self harm is an addiction that must be treated like any other addiction. If left untreated, a self harm addiction will, at the very least, mentally and emotionally destroy the individual and, at the worst, will end up instilling suicidal thoughts and could possible take their life. So, for those who know someone who is self harming, do not let it go. Do not dismiss it as a passing occurrence because it might very well end

Michael Kibler

up killing that person. Instead, treat it with the seriousness and gravity it deserves and seek out help for the individual.

I believe that there are two main types of self harm based on what the individual wants the self harm to do; hidden and seen. Hidden is the most common type of self harm. The individual does not want anyone to see what they have done and it is strictly therapeutic for them. The vast majority of my episodes were hidden. The individual will go to great lengths to cover up the self harm. They will lie to hide the fact that they were self harming. If the individual is accused of self harm, they will become very defensive. Then there's seen. This type of self harm is meant to be seen by someone or a group of people. It usually is a name or word, but can also be a shape or picture. I only preformed this type once. I was dating a very abusive girl and, in order to show my feelings for her, I carved her name into my arm with a razor blade. This type of self harm can be likened to a sort of therapeutic tattooing. The seen self harm is always very methodically planned and carried out. Sometimes the individual won't even care who sees it. What they are trying to do is to send a message. It can be considered a silent cry for help and is a cry for help that must not be ignored. Both types are equally destructive and should be addressed right away.

There are many things that can start a self harming episode. It could be as significant as a death of someone close, or as insignificant as a smile not returned by the cashier at the local grocery store. I can even recall several instances in which I

14

cut for no other reason than to get that endorphin high. When a person starts to self harm for that reason, that's when the addiction is in full force. That's also when the person needs help the most. When the motivation for self harming is the actual act of self harming, then there are virtual no limits or restrictions on what the individual is willing to do to themselves to get that pain. They will do whatever it takes to make them feel better, including more dangerous forms of self harm. And, by having a self harm addiction, the doors are opened to other forms of self medicating addictions such as drug abuse, alcoholism, and overeating. It is far more strenuous and difficult to deal with multiple addictions than it is to deal with a single one. Understanding what motivates an individual to self harm is key in eventually getting them to quit and, by doing so, having them be able to live a better, healthier life.

RECOGNITION

For those who are concerned that someone you know is engaged in self harming, there are different warning signs that you should look for. Probably the biggest indicator is the person's environment. Observe what kind of music they listen to, what kind of shows they watch, what kind of things they read, and who they surround themselves with. If they are constantly immersing themselves in things promoting self harm and continuously with people who self harm, then they are at a higher risk for self harming.

And, believe it or not, there are those out there who actually advocate for self harm. These are the people who glorify self harm as a type of alternative therapy that helps those who practice it. In truth, most of these people are probably individuals who self harm and do not want to quit so they come up with faulty reasons and logic for why they should carry on with their addiction. Any work, written or otherwise, produced by these individuals should be avoided at all cost, as all that it does is to help rationalize self harm to those who come into contact with it. The ultimate goal of an individual who is self harming should be to eventually be able to lead a life free of that addiction, not to rationalize self harm and let it continue to destroy their life.

We are all products of our environments and if that environment is a negative one, so too will our character be inclined to be negative. Self harm must be taught to an individual; it is not natural to harm one's own body in order to feel good. If that teaching can be removed before it takes hold then there is a chance that the individual might not self harm in the first place, which is ultimately the best case scenario.

Another warning sign is the types of clothing they wear. Chances are they will do their best to cover up the areas where the harm themselves. I dated several cutters, many of my friends self harmed, I listened to songs about self harm, and I always wore long sleeve shirts and a watch to avoid detection; I was about as stereotypical as an individual could get when it came to being a cutter.

If you notice that an individual meets these criteria, calmly ask them about it. If you do not feel you can approach them in a calm, cool, and collected state, talk to someone you trust about it or contact a professional. It is important to not be aggressive with a potential self harmer, as they will feel cornered and might become aggressive themselves. The best thing to do is to be sympathetic about what they are going through, even if you have never experienced it. This will help the individual get to a point where they can trust the people they need to get them to quit. If you make this first step a bad experience, the individual will be more reluctant and hesitant to trust others in the future and that will definitely impede their ability to heal later on.

If an individual is engaging in self harm, they should tell someone they trust about it. Many fear that they will end up in a psychiatric ward if they disclose that they are self harming. This is not true. My own therapist sees several individuals who self harm and they are not in any sort of institute. An individual can only be admitted to a place like that if they are a danger to themselves or others. Chances are the individual is neither and, as such, hospitalization is the last thing anyone wants them to experience. Many also fear rejection and disregard about their addiction. If the individual goes to a qualified professional the very opposite will happen; they will be accepted and helped with kind and understanding treatment. The individual should never be afraid of going to see somebody about their addiction. That is the best and fastest way to be healed from their affliction. Therapists and psychiatrists are trained to help with these sorts of things. Their number one priority is the treatment and healing of the individual. These are the best people that the individual can go to for help. If they are not ready to take that step, they should go to someone they trust. Whether it is a peer, co-worker, or a friend, telling someone about their self harm addiction will get a large amount of stress of the individual's mind and, at the very least, can set things in motion to get them the help they both need and deserve.

Just because an individual self harms does not mean that they are in any way mentally ill. More often than not, it means that they lack healthy ways of dealing with unpleasant thoughts, feelings, or situations. Labels, like crazy or insane, are not to be used because they simply are not accurate. Unfortunately there are many out there who do describe self harmers using such labels. Just as they label others, I label them as ignoramuses; these are the people whose words ring out hollow, yet sting all the same. They are to be kept away from the individual as much as possible during the individual's treatment. All it takes is one cruel word or phrase to set the individual back weeks or months in the healing process. Instead, surround the individual with people who love and support them. This will greatly increase their chances of successfully fighting off their self harm addiction sooner.

There is no avoiding it; idiots exist in this world. The ignorant who degrade and put down others because their victims are different from themselves are truly a horrendous kind. Everyone knows who I am talking about. No matter where I go I am always running into them. The way I handle them is by knowing in my heart that I am a better and stronger person than they make me out to be. Anyone who deals with a self harm addiction and chooses to fight it is better in every way than the stupid who poke fun at their vice. That is what the individual must remember. If the individual lets what has been said to them get to them, then the idiots have won. That is the last everyone else wants to happen. So when the individual encounters these types of people (I say people with the same enthusiasm that I say the Nazis were people), they should hold on tightly to the truth; that the individual is fighting against something that the ignoramus could not even imagine in their worst nightmare.

For those who are considering self harm, but have never tried it, a word of advice; don't. If you feel pressured to do so by anyone of anything, do what you can to remove yourself from that temptation. If you feel like that isn't working, contact a professional and seek help. Messing with this sort of thing is like playing with fire; eventually you're going to get burned. A life where you need to hurt yourself in order to even make it through the day is not a very good one to live.

Prevention is the best cure. If an individual shows signs of potentially becoming a self harmer then all reasonable efforts should be made to extinguish the fire before the spark even catches. Anything that encourages self harm must go. If the individual has depression, seek out help for them. The best kind of an addiction is an absent one and this holds true for self harm. By stopping the idea of self harm in its tracks, the individual and those around them have essentially eliminated 99% of the work associated with handling a self harm addiction. If the idea of self harming is allowed to grow into actual behavior, then much hard work is ahead of everyone involved.

When it has been established that an individual is engaging in self harm, there are several facts that must be recognized both by the individual and those wishing to help him or her. Without establishing these facts, the road to recovery will almost certainly be unnecessarily difficult.

First, and probably most importantly, both parties must understand that self harm is a legitimate addiction. To many of those who do not practice self harm, it might not seem like a legitimate addiction because it is so counterintuitive that a person can get addicted to pain. However this is simply not true. Self harm is a very real addiction just as much as alcoholism and overeating are addictions. Some people use self harm to handle life the same way that some people use alcohol or food to handle life. What it all boils down to is that these sorts of addictions create a mask to hide from life's problems. Self harm can also be considered a form of self medication, as the individual who practices it is using it to bring about good feelings via artificial means. If anything, self harm could even be considered to be worse, as the self harmer can practice their addiction virtually any time or anywhere the urge strikes them. Those who do practice self harm and do not see it as an addiction are definitely in denial. In order to be able to rid themselves of this vice, everyone involved must admit the seriousness and reality of this addiction. Only after that can lasting help be administered and accepted.

But at what point does self harm become an addiction. It varies slightly from person to person, but a good litmus test that I use is if an individual needs self harm to feel normal then, chances are, they are addicted. But if anyone is self harming on a regular basis, it needs to be investigated. Now I understand that we all experiment and try things out; I get it. Things happen and we might sometimes do things we regret later on. If someone just tries it once, or even a few times, but does not persist, then that person does not have to worry about having tried it (though if they had a reason to try it in the first place, that probably needs to be examined.) As long as the individual does not feel a need to self harm, then all is well.

Another thing that has to be realized is that self harm is a behavior that must end. There are counter arguments for letting self harm persist. They are mostly from the bias of those who practice it. These arguments very closely follow the logic of the argument for the legalization of marijuana in that it supposedly is very safe and that it only helps those who do it, or that there are no valid reasons to stop. Risks of severe infections and bleeding aside, there is an aspect of self harm that these arguments always fail to cover; consequences. Self harm is usually used as a distracter for an individual's problems, but can never solve said problems. All it does it to mask what may be serious issues. And when a person always falls back on methods that hide problems instead of dealing with them, they turn into a loaded gun ready to fire off at any moment. When that individual is faced with a situation that they cannot hide from, it is very likely that that individual will act, at the very least, in a counterproductive manner and, at the worst, in a potentially deadly manner. Self harm does not solve any problems but, rather, it constructs a temporary mask to hide from the problems.

There are many good reasons to stop self harming. The

increase in quality of life is one of the better incentives to quit. All that anxiety goes away about your life's problems because, instead of distracting yourself from them, you would be actually dealing with and resolving them. You also don't have to worry about being caught and sent to a mental institute (which is not a place that you want to go to.) Then there's all that grief you spare the people that love and care about you because, believe it or not, there are people who do love and care about you and it hurts them to see you like this. For these reasons, self harm is most certainly a behavior that must be corrected.

Anyone can self harm. I was a very outgoing person when I was still cutting and I always appeared happy. No one suspected that underneath my cheerful disposition lurked a wreck of a broken teenager. As self harm is a coping strategy as much as it is an addiction, individuals who do engage in it can outwardly give the appearance of being perfectly alright, while being a shattered mess within. This is because they use self harm to hide from their problems and can fool those around them into thinking that they are fine. Self harming extends throughout all walks of life. I, as a tribute to my love of horses, always don western attire; I dress like a cowboy. For many, a guy who dresses like that would be one of the last people who would be suspected of self harming. Yet I would cut myself nearly every day. Stereotyping has its uses, but not when dealing with self harm. An individual does not need to be dressed in all black and have chains and dark makeup on to self harm, nor must they fit into a strict set of social guidelines to do so either. I know of preteens who self harm as well as adults in their 40s who self harm. I know both guys and girls who self harm. This addiction reaches into every corner of society. If they show signs of being of self harmer, then that needs to be looked into.

If a person knows that an individual is, or possibly is, self harming and is considering letting the issue go, that person should definitely try their best to resolve the issue. This is especially true for those under 18 years of age who want to preserve their friendship with an individual who may be self harming. If left unchecked, a self harm addiction can last an individual's entire life and nobody benefits from that scenario. So if the individual is under 18, do them a favor and get them help. It is far easier to deal with the addiction in the earlier stages of progression. Since the average individual's brain is not fully developed until their mid to late 20s, a self harm addiction may not be fully incorporated into their psyche at this point and it will be much less difficult to treat and heal the individual than if they were to seek help later on in their life. Plus they are still under the authority of their parents and, at the very least, they can be exposed to a wider variety of help whether they want it or not. Unwanted treatment is still treatment and every advantage helps tremendously when dealing with self harm.

It is far better to lose a friend and save a life than to lose a friend and a life. Even if they end of hating the person for the rest of their life, the individual will get exposure to the help they need and will have a much better chance of getting healed than if they were to go without the help. Several of my friends and peers turned me in all throughout the time I was cutting. I specifically recall a time when I was cutting myself in class under my desk and a few girls saw what I was doing and told the teacher what I had done after class. When I carved my ex-girlfriend's name into my arm, my friend turned me in to the school counselor when she saw the scars. I resented and rejected those people because I viewed it as a massive betrayal. As time went on, however, I started to look at them as more of my true friends than those who had idly sat by and done nothing to get me help.

In order for any real progress to be made towards leading a self harm free life, the individual absolutely must have the honest desire to stop. Without that, nothing will be accomplished. The reason I didn't stop cutting after my first visit to a psychiatric institute was because I didn't want to stop. I enjoyed it and felt no need to quit one of the few sources of happiness in my life at the time. It was not until I decided that I wanted to rid myself of that vice that I finally put in the time and effort it took to quit. This holds true with everyone suffering from a self harm addiction; they need to be motivated to quit.

There are many out there who do not want to quit. They want to keep going because they are so addicted to self harm that they feel like they cannot stop. There are also those individuals who don't want to stop because they enjoy it and see no reason to quit. No one can force them to stop self harming. All that will do is make them dig their heels in and refuse to cooperate and ignore any help offered to them. Only when the individual truly wants to stop self harming will they invest in an addiction free future. Until then, the best anyone can do for them is to encourage them to accept the help offered to them. Let them know that things will get better once they choose to quit self harming. You can lead a horse to water, but you can't make them drink. You can offer them the cooling waters of freedom, but only they can choose to drink.

HOW TO HEAL

The first step on the path to healing is to remove any potential sources of temptation from the self harmer. Anything the individual can use to hurt themselves should be removed from their daily environment until the addiction is under control. The less opportunities for a person to hurt themselves the better. At this stage in the game, the addiction should be stopped dead in its tracks before it gets any worse. And it will get worse if left untreated. Make sure to check the areas of the individual's body where they were known to self harm at least once a day to discourage any more self harm. For me, this meant my parents examined my arms daily where I used to cut the most for many months before I could be trusted to not self harm. The main concern here should be the safety of the self harmer; stability is the first priority. The deeper problem solving and motivations behind the self harm should be secondary at this point.

If the individual has multiple preferred methods of self

harm then all efforts should be made to keep them constantly occupied during their treatment. This will help considerably to keep them clean from self harm throughout treatment. While it is not possible to take away every single source of self harm away from the individual, the main objects that the individual used to self harm should be disposed of if possible. When I was cutting, I actually grew emotionally attached to anything that I used to cut myself with. I associated those objects and cutting with feelings of happiness and relief. Chances are most individuals are the same way. That is why it is best to permanently remove those specific objects that the individual self harmed with. If they were to happen across those same objects again the individual could very well go into relapse. I was working at a farm one day when I was about 4 or 5 months clean and came across a razor blade laying on the ground. It was the same type that I used to cut myself with. Instantaneously the urge to cut hit me like a ton of bricks and my fiancée had to throw it away for me because I was too tempted to cut myself with it. Memories and associations are not to be trifled with, especially when dealing with this sort of addiction.

In some instances, the individual might only reveal their addiction when they harm themselves so greatly as to need professional medical attention, such as cutting too deeply or burning too much skin off. I have heard true horror stories of self harmers going to the hospital for their self inflicted wounds only to be met with contempt from the hospital staff and, in some cases, even fail to receive standard treatment for their wounds like not receiving anesthetics for stitches. Just because an injury is the result of self harm does not mean it should be treated inferiorly. If anything, people should do their best to treat the individual with as much care as possible because, if this is the first time that their addiction is out in the open, the way people react to their addiction will make a lasting first impression. This could greatly impact the individual's attempt at healing, so every attempt should be made to make the individual's first glimpse at other people's reaction to their addiction as positive as possible. Otherwise, all those that are treating the individual are doing is to present yet another road block on the already difficult road to recovery.

Finding a therapist with experience in treating self harm is important for ensuring the success of the individual. Every person responds to therapy differently, so it is good to quickly find out what kind of the therapy that the individual takes to the most. For me, one-on-one counseling sessions with the occasional family session worked best. For others, group therapy might be a good option. Just as everyone learns differently, everyone heals differently. Having a treatment plan hand-tailored to the individual's exact needs and requirements will aid quite a lot in healing them. I had one friend who used to cut herself that stopped when her friends would slap her wrists every time she would self harm. This type of tough love is obviously not recommended for every individual. But, for some, being slightly more aggressive might actually aide the healing process as it did in my friend. It all depends on the individual.

I am a huge advocate of having the individual's friends and family playing an active role in the treatment plan. When I first tried to quit cutting I failed miserably because I did not set up a good support system. I tried to take my addiction on as a one man operation and it did not work at all. The reason was because it was simply too much for me to handle. I had no outside encouragement, nor did I have anyone to talk to about my struggle. I isolated myself, therefore I killed my healing. Once I started to open myself up to others, I found that I could more easily start to heal.

Now there are those who believe that hospitalization should be the first step. I disagree. All that does is stress the individual out. And, chances are, they will be more inclined to self harm in a stressful, unfamiliar environment than in one which they are comfortable in. People argue that it provides a safe environment to keep the individual from self harming. However, if an individual truly has their heart set on self harming, nothing short of a straight jacket will prevent them from doing so. That is why a psychiatric institute should be used only as a last resort, or if the individual becomes a threat to themselves or those around them.

In my 2 hospitalizations I have had fairly awful experiences. I felt trapped and alone. I was constantly worried about my personal safety and sanity. It was like being a bird trapped in a cage. I lost a good 15 pounds during my 8 day stay at the first ward off of my already lean 150 pound frame. There was no physical or mental stimulation for me to engage in, and certainly no truly helpful coping mechanisms for me to take part in. I had another guy try to take advantage of my weakened state by trying to put his hand down my pants among other things. I did not take a shower at all during my first stay for fear of being raped. What I remember most about the first stay is a lot of yelling and cursing from the other patients as well as the staff and the frequent fights. Spare the individual of all these horrific experiences if at all possible by avoiding psychiatric institutes. I am not saying that all institutions are bad. In fact my second stay at a different hospital was quite beneficial; the staff was much more supportive and the help offered went much farther. If an individual must be hospitalized, make sure adequate research is done on the different locations to make sure they don't experience the same sort of situations that I went through at my first visit to a psychiatric hospital. You're trying to help them; not make them worse.

The next step should be to get rid of anything that encourages or glorifies self harm. The last thing the individual needs is conflicting messages. If it puts self harm in a positive light, it needs to go. This includes music, propaganda, clothing, and even friends who encourage it. It may stress out the individual temporarily, but will greatly aide them long term in their battle against their addiction.

This will be a very rough time for the individual who, up until recently, was a self harmer. Depending on how much the individual engaged in self harm prior to being cut off from it, there will be some level of detoxification once the individual is cut off. During this detoxification, the person will greatly vary in both emotional and mental states and it is very important to remain supportive throughout all the highs and lows. The individual will be greatly tempted to self harm and will probably attempt it somehow using whatever methods he or she can come by. Persistence in remaining strong, even when the individual is not, is extremely important. If the individual seems unusually calm at any point at this stage, it might become necessary to check more areas of their body than are usually examined, as they might have started to self harm on a new area. The individual will more than likely be very resistant to this idea regardless of whether they are actually harming a new area; if they are not engaging in self harm in a new area they will view this as an unnecessary breech of privacy and, if they are harming a new area, they will be afraid of being caught. In either instance it is important to not back down despite what they say or do. Those who are trying to help must keep in mind that everything they are doing are for the individual's own good, whether the individual recognizes it or not. If it turns out that the individual has been harming in a new area, then that new area must also be checked on a regular basis. Having a strong support system is crucial for the success of the individual. Reassurance is also big part of the detoxification process. Letting the person know that things will get better will help the person along in this phase. Keeping a running tally of time since their last self harm episode can be very encouraging to the individual; it gives them something measurable to mentally weigh their success.

The longer an individual self harmed, the harder it will be to shake off the bonds of their former addiction. That is because the habits of engaging in self harm are embedded into an individual's subconscious and the more that individual self harmed, the more it was engrained into their mind. I had a relatively short-lived addiction at around 2 years. I know of individuals who have self harmed for the majority of their lives. These are the individuals who have the hardest time quitting just because of how long they've been self harming. That is why it is extremely important to eradicate this behavior from a given individual as soon as possible. The longer it lasts, the harder it is to get rid of it.

Medication is something that should also be considered at some point if the individual is having too much difficulty managing their emotions. Some people will probably be very resistant to medications because they might see it as cheating or as a weakness; I know I fought against the idea of medication. However, medications are simply another weapon in the fight against feeling bad. Just because an individual takes a medication does not mean that they are worth any less. It means that they need some extra help. Believe me when I say that every bit of help goes a long way when fighting something as serious as this. That is why it is prudent to listen to the advice of professionals if medication is recommended.

Now if, by some means, the individual does manage to self harm before the detoxification phase is complete (or during any point in the healing process), do not give up hope. As humans we are designed to make mistakes and learn from them. I personally relapsed several times before I finally quit for good, using my failures as learning opportunities to apply towards my eventual quitting. Remaining calm and regrouping is the best strategy for ensuring future success. Remember to think in the long term; everyone's journey to a life free of self harm is different. Some are filled with more obstacles than others. Just because an individual may not progress as fast as he or she would like does not mean that they will never reach their goal. There are many paths to a single destination. Some people just happen to take the scenic route.

With that in mind, the use of positive reinforcement can be very effective in giving the individual incentive to stop. By setting goals, in the form of time gone without an episode, and rewarding those goals with certain privileges, the individual will be able to have some tangible indicator of their progress. In my own case, my parents took away my cell phone when I was hospitalized the first time and told me that if I went three months without cutting that I could earn my phone back. This gave me something to look forward to, especially during the struggles associated with detoxification. The individual should be given as many reasons to quit as possible in order to ease their journey to a self harm free life.

A method that never failed to keep me from cutting was keeping a cutting journal. Whenever I felt like cutting, I would pour out a stream of consciousness onto its pages. Every dark thought I had regarding hurting myself, along with the occasional sketch, would be written down in red ink. It was a very cathartic method of prevention for me for several reasons. First of all, because no one was allowed to read it, I could put down whatever I wanted. This allowed all the bad thoughts and ideas to drain out from my mind, rather than influence me to self harm. Privacy is a big detail with any sort of self harm journal. It allows the individual to have full rein over their thoughts and, by doing so, allows them to purge those ideas that are undesirable. That is why it is very important to allow the individual to have his or her privacy with their journal. Another aspect of the self harm journal is that it allows the writer to see what triggers self harm episodes and, until they learn how to deal with the triggers, avoid them as much as possible. While the self harm journal may contain really dark thoughts, they are completely harmless because of the fact that those thoughts are no longer within the individual's consciousness and are on the pages of the journal instead.

There are some people who may prefer to express their negative feelings in a medium other than words. It might take the form of artwork, crafts, music, or anything that gets the destructive tendencies out of the individual's mind and into a tangible expression. It does not matter how the emotional purge happens. The purpose of this exercise is not to evaluate the work being produced but, rather, to allow the individual a method to release their harmful feelings in a way that does not harm them. In fact, it would probably be counterproductive to have the work produced by the individual looked at by anyone else but the individual. The reason for this is that the individual might not want to express some of the darker thoughts and feelings that the individual is feeling due to a fear of being judged by those assessing their work. In order for this technique to be fully and effectively cathartic, the individual cannot hold back any of the negativity inside their mind. That is why it is probably best to allow the individual complete freedom and privacy when composing any type of cutting journal, written or otherwise. It might even be productive for the individual to personally destroy the journal when they feel they are ready to part with it. For me, seeing my cutting journal consumed in flames provided an additional release on top of what was written in its pages. Watching what represented hundreds of near-episodes burn into oblivion allowed me to further let go of my addiction and progress my healing.

In order to keep the person from focusing on their desire to self harm, it is necessary to replace that desire to hurt themselves with another, positive habit; a distracter. It can take the form of nearly anything. For some, it may be intense exercise like running or weight lifting. For others, it might take the form of intense mental stimulation such as reading or puzzle solving. It might even be as simple as exposure to something that they hold a true passion for. My personal distracter from self harm was horses. I have been a dedicated equestrian since I was six years of age and horses always brought me great joy. So, for my experiences with detoxification, being around horses would always soothe my troubled mind. Anything positive that gets the person's mind away from harming themselves is a step in the right direction. Unfortunately, what can end up happening is replacing one addiction with another. That is why it is prudent to be careful about the way a distracter is introduced to the former self harmer. If those attempting to help try to completely immerse the person in whatever is acting as the distracter, then what happens is that the distracter is no longer distracting, rather it is becoming a substitute for self harm and no matter how harmless the substitute is, too much of a good thing is still too much. This causes problems further down the road when attempts are made to have the person be self fulfilling, as they will no longer be addicted to self harm but, rather, a whole new habit that must end up being broken. There is no such thing as a healthy addiction.

A technique that many people use to prevent a self harming episode is to draw or write something on where they most frequently self harm on their bodies. The purpose of this is to give the individual a sort of "last chance" to ward off a particular episode before it can begin. Usually when an individual is about to self harm, they will examine the area on which they most often do so to see specifically where they will self harm. If there is a significant drawing or word in between them and their skin, it can deter the individual from self harming. At the very least it can make the individual think twice about self harming. I really wish I knew about this method when I was still actively cutting. I always would examine my arm thoroughly before I would cut myself and to have something in ink scribed there probably would have done me a great deal of good.

There are those who advocate for distracters that involve pain or discomfort that leave no permanent scars, such as squeezing ice cubes or consuming hot sauce. This method of distraction is counterproductive, however, as all it does is feed into the individual's addiction to the good feelings brought about by pain by providing them with the very pain they both want to experience and need to avoid. It is important to remember that the main reason that individuals self harm is to experience pain in order to, in turn, experience positive feelings. Allowing individuals to experience non-scarring pain is still allowing them to succumb to their addiction. Allowing them to succumb to their addiction may severely hinder their healing and that will lead only to frustration. It is important to look at things in terms of long term healing, as well as short term healing. The individual needs to be as safe and as comfortable as possible in the short term but, at the same time, energy should be devoted towards maintaining perspective on the situation at all times. What sets back the individual temporarily may well be good for them in the long run. A balance must be struck between the two for the fastest road to healing to be achieved.

The individual's environment must be kept as clean as possible of anything that could start an episode. This will be a temporary setup, as eventually the individual must learn how to be self fulfilling and deal with external problems without reverting to self harm. Balance is a crucial part of dealing with a self harm addiction. Weighing safety versus healing can be very tricky, but safety should always take priority. There will always be time to work on emotional healing after the individual has calmed down.

Do everything possible not to make the individual feel trapped. Let them have access to any healthy friendships and relationships. Any friends that are supportive and do not take part in unhealthy habits should be allowed to communicate with the individual. If there is a significant other in the individual's life that is the same way, let the individual have full access to them. If, on the other hand, you had a relationship like mine in which the other party encouraged self harm and/or other harmful ideas, it is probably best to seek help for the other person or, if that person refuses to accept help, to discourage or restrict the relationship. It will definitely sting the individual emotionally for a while in the short term, but in the long term, will save them a whole lot of grief and suffering. My now (thankfully) ex-girlfriend was a cutter and had no intentions of stopping. When I needed her the most, in my first visit to a mental institution, she abandoned me, moved on, and eradicated me from her life. And while it hurt very much at the time, I reflect back on that as a positive occurrence in my past in which a negative force was removed from my life. On the reverse, if the individual's friend/significant other is willing to accept help, then by all means they should be allowed to communicate. Tough times are always easier to undergo when we can relate to someone close to us.

Should the individual communicate that they feel like self harming, remain calm and ask them why they feel that way. By finding out the source of the negative feelings, those trying to help the individual can address it and help the individual through whatever is bothering them. It is extremely important to keep all emotions in check when attempting to provide help for the individual. Those who are trying to help must remain steadfast with their emotions, otherwise any drastic feelings will translate down to the individual and that is never a good thing considering that the individual is not good at managing their feelings in the first place. There should be a good example set for the individual for how to solve a problem rather than reacting to it.

If those trying to aid the individual feel that their actions are inadequate for helping the individual, they should seek out a professional. A school student would seek out the school counselor or a trusted teacher just like an adult would suggest a therapist for a peer. No one will benefit from actions that do not really help. If those trying to help truly want to see the individual get better but don't know how to make that happen, it is best to seek out a good therapist with experience in treating self harm addictions. It might not feel right at first having the situation taken out of their control, but it will help everyone involved further down the road to healing.

I also recommend those affected by someone with a self harm addiction seek out help as well. There will more than likely be quite a bit of stress on them and it pays to invest time in help that can then be imparted to the individual later on. There is absolutely no point in attempting to help an individual when the person trying to help is lacking the very thing they are trying to instill. There is a saying I like that applies to this instance: "You need to help yourself before you can help others." Only when a person is fully healed themselves can they start to heal others.

Towards the end of the detoxification period the individual will start to calm down considerably. They will be less prone to extreme outbursts and will be more inclined to accept help from those around them. Take advantage of this change in attitude by congratulating them of their progress and start to give them the tools they need to be self fulfilling. This is where positive reinforcement really can make a difference on an individual's progress. By rewarding the individual somehow, they will start to view not self harming in a better light. I know that after my three months were up I was ecstatic to get my phone back. That made my success at going that long without cutting all the more sweet. All those little victories soon add up into a larger triumph that will endure for the rest of the individual's life.

But what is self fulfillment? I have mentioned self fulfillment a couple of times already in a positive way. That is because it is a very good state of mind to be in especially for those who have suffered from a self harm addiction. Self fulfillment is when an individual does not require anything external to be content; their main source of happiness comes from within. They need nothing but themselves to be truly happy. This is what everyone suffering from a self harm addiction should strive for because, once reached, self fulfillment eliminates the reasons to engage in self harm. Another part of self fulfillment is the ability to handle a given situation without falling back on something that merely masks the issue at hand. Being able to deal with a problem is a skill that, once learned, can be applied throughout one's entire life. It is also something that makes self harm obsolete to anyone, because if a given person is able to solve problems then there will be no need to hide from them.

Once the detoxification process has ended, the individual will be much calmer and should be open to deeper help. They will no longer be in imminent danger of harming themselves and can be trusted to be by themselves more often. However, just because they are more stable, does not mean that the people trying to help can let their guard down. If the individual self harms again, the whole detoxification process must begin anew. Keeping the individual clean of self harm will help in the long run by giving them something to look back on with pride as they observe their progress take shape.

Seize the opportunity by beginning to ask questions about the individual's self harming habits. Thorough, but gentle, inquiry should be made at this point. Find out as much as possible about what caused the first episode, what usually causes episodes to occur, where episodes happen the most, how they carry out episodes, and anything else that those trying to help deem relevant. Those attempting to help the individual should be looking for any patterns in the individual's self harm habits. Once identified, these patterns can be looked at to find out the main cause or causes of the individual's addiction.

Talking about their addiction will actually act as a cleansing catharsis for the individual. Relating facts about their self harm habits should not be discouraged for fear of relapsing, but encouraged to keep from relapsing. It follows the same principle as the self harm journal previously mentioned. When those bad thoughts and memories are allowed to build up and stew inside an individual, nothing good can be accomplished. But when those things are released in a safe environment, they become harmless ideas of the past. That is why I would talk about cutting whenever I was under stress. It wasn't that I was relapsing (as my parents often feared); it was just my way of undoing my internal tension. Even writing this book is quite therapeutic for me. Keeping bad memories and ideas locked up inside is the very worst thing an individual can do.

I would also show my friends the scars on my wrist, not because I was seeking attention, but because sharing my pain with another helped to keep me calm. That is often the case for self harmers; they are not out for attention. They are usually trying to relieve some of the enormous pressure they are feeling not only from their addiction, but from their lives as well. This type of behavior is usually dismissed as attention grabbing when, in all reality, it is nothing of the sort. I have never encountered an individual who self harmed for the purpose of getting attention. While there are those out there who do that, they are certainly the minority. For the most part, those who self harm and show others their wounds are trying to get rid of stress and are not trying to get noticed. This is apparent by who they choose to show and the manner in which they do so. In my own case, I would only show those I trusted not tell anyone about my addiction and I would explicitly ask them not to inform anyone about it.

When the most common causes of the individual's episodes are recognized, that is when the individual should start to work through being able to handle those triggers when they arise in his or her life. My most frequent trigger was other peoples' relationships. As a high school student, I was used to seeing couples around the school on a daily basis. All it took was for me to see them holding hands to trigger a cutting episode. That is because I was in and out of horrid relationships throughout my junior and senior years and I envied those couples' happiness. All I cared about at the time was being in a happy relationship. It was not until I found self fulfillment that I could finally have a healthy and happy relationship.

Do not attempt to bury the past prematurely when helping the individual. If they try to forget about what has happened to them before those memories are resolved, then nothing will have been accomplished. The point of healing is to heal, not to hide. And, chances are, they will be at a higher risk for relapse because those triggers that reside in the individual's memories will still be active. Instead, talk about those triggers as often as the individual can bear and explore them. The purpose is to expose the individual to as much of what triggers their episodes as possible in an environment in which they cannot engage in self harm. That way, instead of relying on their addiction to protect them, they are forced to learn how to deal internally with whatever is bothering them. And it really is an internal struggle for the individual, as for however long they were self harming they were without ways to solve their life's problems.

An idea that I would highly recommend would be to have the individual talk to someone who has successfully ridded themselves of a self harm addiction. I was talking to my step-father one day about how I wanted to help others who struggle with a self harm addiction just like I did, and he said that I had about as much right to speak about how to quit self harm as an alcoholic does to speak about how to quit drinking. I paused, thought for a few moments, and replied, "I quit cutting; therefore I know how to quit." That is the only time I remember beating my father in a difference of opinion. I fully believe that, if you have accomplished something, that gives you every right to be able teach others how to do the same. This applies to those who have quit self harming. They have real life experience and they know what works and does not. In this way, they have an advantage over the book knowledge found in the minds of those therapists and psychiatrists who deal with this sort of addiction in that experience is the best teacher and nothing can top practical knowledge.

Only when the individual can talk about every single

trigger in their life comfortably with another can the past be laid to rest. I tried so hard for so long to undo the mistakes of my past only to be met with constant disappointment and frustration. It was not until I realized that I needed to set my sights to the future that I was able to live a happier and better life. The individual must realize that they cannot change what has come and gone. Encourage them to live in the present, look forward to the future, and learn from the past. Everyone makes mistakes; that is what makes us human. What defines us is not what we did in our past; rather it is how we apply past mistakes to contribute towards future successes.

When the individual is able to discuss the things that would trigger their episodes, it is time to move on to teaching them how to deal with those triggers and any other potential triggers that they might encounter. Impart to them different methods of problem solving that best suits them. Teach them how to tackle life's problems instead of hiding from them. Find out the best way for them to handle adverse situations.

It is very important to have a fallback plan for when the individual feels like self harming again because they will feel the urge to do so at some point. Whenever I feel like cutting, I talk to my fiancée (to whom this book is dedicated to) and look at all of our pictures and think back on all of my fond memories with her. What the individual needs to do is to find a few things that are almost always available, easy to explore, and emotionally and mentally soothing. In this day and age of cell phones, the good memories of the past are almost always accessible in the form of pictures. The individual should keep many pictures of their favorite experiences or activities readily available for when the urge to self harm. Another good form of distracter is exercise. I try to run at least 5 miles a day to keep my stress levels down and to keep healthy. I also ride and train horses almost every day. Find an exercise or sport that the individual enjoys and encourage them to make it a large part of their life. Not only will that keep the individual from self harming, but it is also good for their physical health.

I have mentioned my passion for horses a few times throughout this book. Both my fiancée and I are avid animal lovers and we both find animals to be extremely therapeutic in even the most stressful of times. Humans have used their animal brethren as companions for tens of thousands of years and, today, there is much exploration being done in the field of animal therapy. Humans are, by nature, social beings, so it only makes sense that we get along so great with other species. When an individual feels like self harming and a sociable animal is an option to pursue, by all means go right ahead and follow it through. I have found it very helpful even to just be in the presence of an animal whenever I'm feeling particularly down. I attribute this to several factors. For one, animals are innocent. They commit no crime other than what is taught to them by an outside source. There is nothing naturally malicious in an animal outside of survival instincts. Maybe being in the vicinity of such purity has a calming effect on us Homo Sapiens. Another aspect is that an animal will almost always show unconditional love towards people who have not hurt it. By taking advantage of this positive energy, the individual might become positive themselves. I always find it difficult to be depressed in the presence of such happiness. Animals are also hypersensitive to our emotions as a result of being around humans for many millennia. This can play a huge part in an individual's healing. Whenever the individual is feeling the urge to self harm, the animal can help to comfort them.

And, if all else fails, have the individual talk to someone they trust. It can be very therapeutic to verbally unload all of that built up stress and anxiety onto sympathetic ears. This goes along with not isolating the individual during any phase of healing. As humans, we are all social creatures who rely on other humans to keep us sane. No person is an island. When I was healing, and even when I was still cutting, talking to my friends would help me tremendously and would even stop my episodes before they happened. The power of a good friend is not to be underestimated.

In fact, it was not until I looked into the eyes of my fiancée and swore to her that I would never cut again that I quit for good. My love for her overshadowed the desire to relapse and made me clean for good. She has been there with me through thick and thin, and I felt it was only right that I honored the promise I made to her to quit. Whenever I feel like taking a razor to my wrist now, I remember my promise to her and go through my coping strategies until the urge passes. That is what ultimately kept me from self harming for good. So if the individual has someone like that in their life, have the individual promise to them that they will stop self harming. The influence of a verbal contract with someone the individual has a true bond with can change the individual's whole life permanently in a good way. Take advantage of this and have the individual make agreements with people they trust. It does not have to be for an infinite length of time. Take it one baby step at a time and go from week to week or month to month, gradually increasing the time the agreements are good for every time a new one is made. Eventually, once the individual is ready, they will be able to make that promise not to self harm indefinitely. That will give them a big incentive to stay clean for the rest of their lives.

Once the individual has made it this far, they are perfectly justified in calling themselves quitted of self harm. They are now self-fulfilling in being happy with themselves from within themselves. They no longer need to hide behind self harm for life's problems. They can solve most of their issues and, when they cannot, the individual now has several tools and strategies that they can use to keep themselves from self harming. Now, more than likely, they will need to be watchful of relapse for the rest of their life. They will need to be careful to ensure that they do not go back to their old vices. They will need to change a few aspects of their life; the people they hang out with, the music they listen to, the thing they watch, etc. But, all things considered, that is a small price to pay for the freedom brought about by a life liberated from self harm.

LIFE AFTER QUITTING

Slowly, time will begin to erase the scars, both physical and mental, of the individual's self harm addiction. Most of my cuts have faded away already. The emotional damages will probably take a little longer to heal; I know I'm still healing from my past. That is why the individual can never truly let their guard down with regards to their past. All it takes is a single cut, burn, or bruise to bring back a flood of traumatic memories to the individual. One day, after I had quit cutting, I was opening a package with a steak knife and nicked my thumb on the blade of the knife. Instantly I remembered how good it felt to cut and, with that remembrance, came all the memoires of my past that I tried so hard to lay to rest. It was like being in the midst of a raging river trying to sweep me away. But I stayed strong and resisted the impulse to relapse. The important thing is to not let these instances influence the individual's actions. The individual should always be aware of their limitations as far as the temptation to relapse goes. Using the things they learned to help them deal with any future problems is paramount in staying clean for good and remaining self fulfilling.

It is very likely that the individual will carry around the burden of those bad memories the rest of their life; such is the nature of an addiction. There will be times where they will be tempted to go back to their old vices. I know I've been tempted plenty of times since I've quit. And it is only natural to feel that way, as we fall back on what we know during times of great stress. That is why the individual must retrain themselves to use their coping strategies instead of masking their problems.

Once the individual is healed, those things that triggered them, as well as anything they used to conduct their self harm with, must be slowly and safely reintroduced to them. The reason for this is because there will be times when the individual is faced with these objects again and they must learn how to handle them. The best way to do this is for the individual to be with a person or persons who are supportive and introduce these objects to the individual. It was not until recently that I was able to hold a razor blade in my hand without feeling tempted to cut myself. The way I got over this was by having my fiancée watch me whenever I handled a blade and take it away from me if I got too focused on it. The purpose here is to disassociate the objects with negative experiences and emotions and associate them with positive experiences and emotions. So, for example, instead of me remembering my cutting episodes whenever I looked at a razor blade, I now remember my fiancée and I scrapbooking together. Replacing negative experiences with positive ones is the key to long-term success.

Like I mentioned earlier, the length of time that a person self harms plays a critical role in the speed of their recovery. It also can dictate how intense the urges will be post-healing and how often they occur. The individual should not get frustrated if they feel like they have the urges too much and too strongly. As time goes on, the urges will begin to fade and become more and more bearable and manageable. Life will have its ups and downs; more urges will come and go. Everyone is different and, as such, everyone heals differently. Healing might take longer for some than for others. What matters is not the quantity of time it takes to heal, but the quality of the healing itself. There are many different paths to healing, but they all lead to a better life. Staying the course and seeing it through to the end is what healing is all about.

I always run into those ignorant people who blow me off as an "emo freak" because of my past. I even had a few friends that turned their backs to me after they found out what I did. I was quite upset over that for a long time until I realized that those types of people are not who I really wanted or needed to have as friends. I am infinitely better off without having them in my life. No doubt those who share my journey will also encounter these people. That's ok. My mother had a saying that I apply to this situation; "People are always entitled to their opinion, no matter how wrong it is." These are the people that I just smile at and move on with my life, because I know that I fought and won against something that they couldn't even imagine. Life is what you make of it and not what other people think of you. You are an individual and your own person. That's what self fulfillment truly is all about; not needing to impress or please anyone but yourself to be happy.

As more time passes, the urges to self harm will become fewer and farther apart. The temptations will grow weaker and the time between them will grow longer. Soon the urges will become more of an annoyance than an actual threat. The number of things that would have been triggers will decrease. Eventually the individual will get to a point where they will go days, weeks, months, and even years without a serious temptation to self harm. There will be small urges here and there, but nothing that the individual is not capable of handling. Fewer things will be found stressful and more things will be found enjoyable. And with all of that comes peace; a true, happy type of inner peace that can only be achieved by being self fulfilling. It is difficult to explain how it feels. For me it is greater than any high brought about by cutting. The best part about it is that it comes from within. I don't need a blade and blood to make me happy; I am happy because I am happy.

HOPE

Since I quit cutting my life has done a complete turnaround. I am a horse trainer, riding instructor, and writer in southern Maryland. I have met the love of my life and we are engaged to be married once our lives stabilize. She is unlike anyone I have ever met in that she is perfect for me. She supports me, takes care of me, treats me right, and loves me. I love her with all my heart and look forward to spending the rest of my life with her. I hope to someday own a horse farm with my amazing future wife. Until then, I will work as a trainer with her.

I also want to help others who have the same addiction as I did. That's why I wrote this book; to help others. But I want to do more. That's why my other major is communications. When I publish this book, I will become a motivational speaker and give clinics to those who practice self harm or know somebody that does. It is becoming more and more prevalent throughout the world and that needs to change.

This book is only the first step in my new journey; my journey to rid the world of this evil vice called self harm. It is a long journey, but a fruitful one. It will not be easy and will probably outlive me, my children, my grandchildren, and all those to come after me. This is a battle that will more than likely span until the end of humanity. While we may never eradicate it from the face of this earth, we can sure put up a nasty fight. If I can help at least one person, then I have succeeded. I know I cannot help everyone, but why should that stop me from trying? Why should it stop us from trying?

Now I am happy; truly happy. I have never been this happy in my entire life. Words fail to describe how complete I am. It's amazing. I went from rock bottom to sky high in under a year. I look back on my life and have trouble believing that I am the same person who used to cut himself every day. In a way, I am not the same person. We share the same body, but not the same personality. The old me was sad, dark, depressed, mean, sour, and incomplete. I am not him. I am happy, energetic, joyous, nice, sweet, and complete. I resemble him only in physical form. Everything else has changed for the better.

For those who practice self harm who think that they will never get better, rest assured that there is always hope. Things will get better; things always get better. Those who practice self harm and overcome it will come out a stronger person and better for it. I look back on my experiences with my addiction as building character. I am thankful that I can use my negative past and turn it into a positive future, not only for myself but for others as well. I want my legacy to be that I helped at least one person realize that there is a better life free from self harm. That is what my aspirations are. In my opinion, what makes a person great is not the quantity of things written about them, it is the quality of they actually accomplished. I could have chosen to try to cover up my past and forget about it, but that doesn't really help anyone. Instead I have opened myself up to the world in an attempt to come to the aid of those who think they are hopeless. My best advice to those who have triumphed over self harm is to do the same. Lend a helping hand to those in need of it. Together we can turn this epidemic into a thing of the past.

I was about as typical a broken teenager as a person could get. My life was shattered as far as I was concerned. I didn't think anyone could sink as low as I did. But, with the help of all the people that love and care about me, I was able to pick myself up off the floor and put the pieces of my life back together. Bit by bit, I started to heal and today I am successful and live a life free of self harm. If you or someone you know self harms, I sincerely hope that this book has given you at least some of the help you needed. If there is one thing that I want you to take away from this book, it is that there is always hope.

ABOUT THE AUTHOR

Michael Kibler was born and raised in Maryland. He started his 2 year long addiction with cutting in his junior year of high school. Today he is clean of self harm and wants to help others do the same.

Proof

Made in the USA
Charleston, SC
27 April 2013